Unique Kids.

Unique Surroundings.

Creative,

"Green",

Budget-Conscious

Ways to Design the Ideal Environment for

Children with Autism and Special Needs

By

Lauren S. Henry

Edited by

P. Daniel Newman

Unique Kids. Unique Surroundings.

ISBN 978-0-557-09413-4

First Printing August, 2009

Contents

Dedication

This book is dedicated to all who have been so selflessly generous and labored along with me allowing my efforts to continue over the past seven years. *With a Brush of Love* was established in June of 2002 and has been the most intense journey of my life thus far.

Thank goodness for the extraordinary people who've agreed to accompany me along the way. Whether for a short time or the full unexpected roller coaster ride, these individuals have made *EVERYTHING* possible.

Molly, Diana, "Marshmallow," Keri, Marty, Jamie, Shary, Monique, Holly, Callie, Bryan, Jonathan, Larry, my selfless, tirelessly supportive and overall "impressive" grandmother and PCC. Phil, who has been there to support and believe in me since the genesis of this company when an idea simply popped into my head: "what if I created a company that...?" By the time I finished the sentence, he was already as excited as I was. He even accompanied me to Home Depot on my very first job, just to make sure I didn't have a paint induced "panic attack"! Since then, he's always been there with an absolute "yes you CAN" in response to almost any and every question I've come up with and has continued to do so every step of the way (doubting oneself was never an option!) A good friend to have around if you're lucky enough to be blessed with one.

Most Importantly, is the "*CAPTAIN* "— My closest friend, confidant, "jack of *every* trade" and all around personal Superhero! (Everyone should have one of those too!) I've been undoubtedly blessed in this area!

My gratitude, spirituality and faith are boundless as the guidance I continue to receive acts as a conscious reminder that I am on MY "right" path regardless of the tumbles and scrapes I may endure along the way, for that I am eternally grateful. (Band-aids are a basic necessity...)

Last, but certainly not at all least, are Mike and Carol, my phenomenally supportive parents, for the examples they've set, the work ethic they've instilled, and the warmth, kindness and generosity of spirit they extend to all those around them. Thank you for teaching me the mantra: "I can do anything I set my mind to as long as I don't give up – push, press, persist, never give in." Having a fiercely independent-minded daughter hasn't always been easy, and that is something I recognize.

I know you will all remain alongside me as **With a Brush of Love** continues to grow, fulfilling all the goals we've discussed and envisioned together! This labor of love is also a tribute to every single one of **YOU!**

For ALL these many reasons, I THANK YOU, LOVE YOU and am grateful I can call you my family and my FRIEND.

Foreword

The term "special needs children" is misleading. Every child is unique, and has needs that are specific to them. Everyone experiences things a little differently. We all have different sensitivities to color, light, sound, taste and touch. As adults, we build our surroundings based on our personal preferences; things that make us feel good. Our children do not have the same power.

We often wonder how to do what is best for our children. How does one make the "right" decision for each individual child? After all, the personality traits and characteristics of one child are rarely identical to our own, or those of their siblings. While there are typically similarities, we are often surprised by our children's natural affinities and interests. They can surprise us even more by the way they think or react. What most people are unaware of is that the way they think and react, focus their attention and absorb information, can be greatly affected by their environment.

Everyone learns in their own way, at their own pace. Just because one child is able to assimilate information in a classroom setting doesn't mean they are more intelligent than another. It simply means they learn differently. They focus their attention and concentration in a way that another child may not. They hear language or absorb writing on a chalkboard or screen in a different way.

Color can have a significant impact on how we learn. Children, even more than adults, are influenced emotionally and intellectually by color. Children learn and retain information longer when color is used in educational material and in the classroom. Approximately eighty percent of the information the brain receives is visual. Color stimulates the visual sense and encourages the retention of information.

To understand how color might be used constructively, it is important to understand the response that color elicits within the typical human being. Keep in mind that there are exceptions to every rule. Not every person responds to color in the same way. However, there are certain generalities that apply to the majority of people, and one of the goals of this book is to share those principles so that they may be utilized to their greatest effect.

Consider your own home. Is there a particular room in which you spend the majority of your time? How does the environment in that room make you feel? Is it soothing? Uplifting? Energizing? There are many factors that contribute to how an environment will affect you. The color, the lighting, the comfort of the furniture, the sound; all these sensory elements impact the emotional effect of the space. Now, consider your child. They are affected profoundly by their environments, but have far less control than you. Special needs, and autistic children in particular, are far more sensitive to sensory stimuli than neuro-typical children, so even more care needs to be given to their surroundings.

Parents can provide a creative environment in the home to inspire imagination and learning. Typically, the use of bright colors in an infant's bedroom seems to be beneficial to the baby's intellectual development. Colorful toys and decor create an environment conducive to both fun and learning. However, when working with special needs and autistic children, the rules often change dramatically.

Color influences mood. Some colors typically induce a comfortable feeling while others can induce the feeling of excitement, energy and stimulation. With special needs and autistic children, these generalities become extremely important. Their tendency to be hyper-sensitive to visual and other sensory stimuli makes it necessary to plan differently. Unfortunately, there are no guidelines that work for all children. Two children with autism could react completely differently to the same color, sound or texture. The solution needs to be personalized for each child, and designed with great care.

In the chapters ahead, we will explore the various factors that should be considered in designing an environment for an individual child. While nothing works for everyone, there are certainly some rules that apply to many, perhaps even most. We will discuss these, as well as ways to determine how to apply them to your child.

As you read this guide of helpful hints, enjoy it, let it inspire you, and always remember to start everything you do

With a Brush of Love.

Chapter 1:

Evaluate Your Child's Needs

Children with autism typically experience an unusually powerful response to sensory stimuli. To them, the experience of daily life can be complete overload. A sound that we might normally tune out could be like a bombardment to their ears. Colorful designs and patterns that we find pleasant could send their minds into overdrive. Everything could be too bright, too loud, too scratchy, and simply too much for them to handle.

Environment for these children is profoundly important. It influences how they feel, how they concentrate, how they communicate, how they sleep, and how they relate to others. All sensory stimuli within your child's space must be considered with a critical eye.

When evaluating your child's needs, try to remain as objective as possible. Whether your child is considered "neuro-typical," has been diagnosed on the autism spectrum, or has been diagnosed with any other condition that may require specific care and attention, determining their individual needs will be a unique journey of discovery. A diagnosis is often just a label; a generality. It provides a guideline, but does not clearly define your child's needs.

Some of us keep journals about our dreams, our feelings, important moments or significant days in our lives. We may journal what we eat and how it affects us, or our sleep patterns. This tool can be very helpful in the process of evaluating your child's needs. Keep a journal of their behaviors: their patterns, chosen activities and communication, both positive and negative. Note where they like to spend their time, what toys they play with, how they react to different objects, places, sights and sounds. Observation is critical. If you pay close attention, you may notice specific causes and effects.

Your child may react in a certain way to a noise, activity around them, bright colors or lights, crowds vs. isolation, music vs. speech, warm colors vs. cool, bright colors vs. soft, textures or colors of foods, clothing, bedding, even every day toiletries. Observe them outside while they interact with nature: dirt, trees, leaves, grass and water. Do they interact better on their own or do they try to involve you in any way? What are they doing when they're the most content? What rooms do they continually gravitate to, and what do those rooms look like? What colors are consistently surrounding them when they are most at ease, or conversely, when they are the most agitated or uncomfortable?

It's important to recognize if and when your child tries to connect with you. Autistic children sometimes do this through unconventional means. When he is hungry, he may open a cabinet containing food that he wants rather than directly ask for it. She may follow you to whatever room you are in and play there, just to be in your presence.

These behaviors can communicate what your child wants or is feeling, but because of the subtlety and indirectness of it, the message can go unnoticed. Recognizing these things can help you understand how to provide a more comfortable environment for your child.

Children are often drawn to particular colors without understanding why. Adults do this as well, though we can usually articulate the reason when asked to consider it. Children may not be able to express that they're scared, sad or excited, but they may gravitate toward particular colors in response to those feelings. For example, they might select a certain color with which to write or draw. They may cling to a particular piece of clothing or a blanket. Both the colors and textures of these items may give them comfort.

Children who are only moderately verbal may have a little trouble putting their exact feelings into words. However, they may be able to describe their feelings more easily by using colors as their guide. You can ask them what kind of day they had or simply how they're feeling. If you guide them by offering them visual choices, they may respond with "dark red" or "bright orange." Perhaps they will relate their feelings by pointing to a color or using a specific color marker or crayon when drawing. They may not have the vocabulary to express their emotions any other way. There are forms of communication other than the spoken word.

More common, and more extreme behaviors, are easier to recognize and comprehend. Many autistic children act out physically when they are frustrated or upset as well as when they're excited and happy. They can hit objects or other people, bang their heads against the wall, or rock back and forth incessantly, sometimes in silence, sometimes vocalizing or even screaming. Then there are those who are withdrawn. They remain apart from others, either watching or simply keeping to themselves. They may be lethargic or inattentive. There are many behaviors that can give you a clear indication that your child may have a unique need. There are also behaviors commonly referred to as "stimming." These are typically repetitive movements that can be either self-stimulating or soothing: rocking, spinning, flapping of hands or arms, etc. Stimming behaviors can also include vocal, tactile (scratching or rubbing) or visual stimuli (fast patterned blinking or squeezing one's eyes shut in an effort to communicate an idea, feeling or experience they want to share.) These behaviors can be a sign of under-stimulation in some children, hypersensitivity in others. In either case, it is helpful to observe the conditions in which a child exhibits stimming behaviors, as this can help reveal environmental elements that are detrimental to the child.

In the simplest terms, children who act out or exhibit aggressive tendencies may need a more soothing, pacifying environment. Children who are withdrawn or lethargic may benefit from a more stimulating environment. Children with attention deficits need an environment that helps them focus. Exactly what will satisfy those needs may not be obvious. Documenting your child's behaviors and observing certain details can help. Note the rooms and places they consistently gravitate toward, and objects, colors or sounds they react to (both positively and negatively). Also pay attention to individuals they want to be near as well as those they wish to avoid. All of these behaviors can help you find the answers. It may be necessary to shift both the way you observe and what you look for. Once you make that shift, you will be well on your way to creating the optimal environment for your child.

Several years ago I painted a mural for a child who was extremely lethargic and withdrawn. The mural, which I referred to as the "energy wall", was bright and extremely stimulating, with various shapes and colors. One of the more unusual concepts within the piece was little bubbles painted on a white background, creating a slight 3-D effect.

A neighbor brought her autistic son, Zach, along with her when she came to see it. Zach was about four years old, very distant and detached. He did not hug or show any sign of affection or emotional connection to his family. After Zach took in the energy wall for a few minutes, he shocked his mother by taking her hand and pulling her toward the wall. He began to trace her finger over the same two bubbles over and over again. He never said anything, but he looked at her and smiled. When his mother stopped to pick him up and hug him, he continued to trace the circles on her clothing and pulled at her until she put him back down and allowed him to continue tracing the bubbles. It was the first time Zach had ever tried to include his mother in his world and share something with her; communicate directly with her. A newfound observation and connection was made between parent and child.

Many parents and caregivers of autistic children understand this experience all too well. Moments like these are very significant for any parent or family member, a reminder that their child is "in there", present and completely whole. They may not be able to express themselves in a way you can immediately relate to, but there are always different ways to foster that kind of growth. Many possibilities exist in order to discover how children will ultimately choose to express themselves, and to learn how to enter their world, at least in some small way.

Chapter 2:

Understand the Purpose of the Space

Before you design the environment of a given room, the first thing you need to do is understand its purpose. This may not be as simple as it seems. A bedroom is the place where we sleep. It's also a sanctuary. It could be a place to play, a place to study, or a place to socialize. Each of these uses may have different design implications.

It's up to you as a parent to decide what the emphasis of the room should be. You may have separate bedrooms and playrooms for your child. You may have an office that doubles as a playroom, or as the room in which your child is expected to study, do homework or have in-home therapies. In order for therapists to be most effective, they need to work in an environment free of distractions. That's no easy task when using a room for multiple purposes.

The reason all these considerations are so important is that the energy of the space needs to be conducive to all its needs. The use of the word "energy" here is not so much a "new age" application, but rather a psychological one. An environment, and all its sensory elements, create a type of energy. Reflect on your own experiences in different environments: offices, waiting rooms, restaurants, friends' homes. As you think of these places, try to recall how you felt upon entering each location, as well as how you felt after you'd been there for a certain amount of time. What design elements did you notice? How did the surroundings make you feel? If you haven't done so in the past, experiment and try it the next time you go somewhere new. Be conscious of these questions as well as your reactions. Most likely, you'll find it to be a very telling and informative experience and you will become much more aware of yourself and what affects you.

One of the most environmentally impactful places people typically go is a restaurant. Have you had a particular dining experience made better or worse due to the atmosphere, or lack thereof? The noise? The lighting? The décor? The music? The comfort of the seats? Let's be honest, very often a dining experience can be improved a great deal beyond the quality of the food or the service. Restaurants often create sensory overload, a perfect example of how the energy of an environment impacts us. Additionally, a large amount of energy is generated by the customers and staff. The environment can make the experience either less or more tolerable simply based on your sensory reactions.

In order to truly understand a space, one must recognize that every object in it affects its energy. Some objects give off energy, some absorb it. This may seem an esoteric concept, but keep an open mind. Every space has a purpose, and in order to fulfill that purpose most effectively, we must design it to have the right kind of energy.

Determining the way a room should be utilized has to do with energy flow, aesthetic appeal, and function. Obviously, one would consider measurement constraints, but there are so many other considerations. Types of lighting and traffic flow are just a couple of examples but happen to be among the most important. Have you ever been in two different homes with the same floor plan and compared how the space was utilized by each resident? Did you feel, to an extent, that the two were entirely different due to the décor and organization? Sometimes it's hard to believe that the exterior shells and architectural layouts are exactly the same.

Some of the more dramatic differences may result from color schemes, patterns or furniture selection. Perhaps you find yourself thinking, "I never would have thought to do that."

Conversely, you might think, "I don't like this at all." Perhaps it feels too stark or closed off. That may be because the design doesn't match your personality, your energy, or a "natural flow" you are comfortable with. (It might also mean the owners have bad taste! But who are we to judge?)

We're all affected by every experience we've had since birth, therefore each of us finds comfort in different environments. Most of us rarely contemplate the reasons we react in certain ways, but when designing a space for your child, this is a very important consideration.

The first step is to understand the purpose of the room so that you can determine the kind of energy it should have. If it has multiple purposes, you'll want to find a balance, and emphasize the uses that are most important. When you recognize the type of energy you want to create, you will be well on your way to designing the ideal environment for you and your child.

There are many aspects to creating a particular type of energy. Color is one of the most significant. Lighting and organization come next. Do you want an open, spacious feeling or do you prefer a cozy, intimate, secure atmosphere? Again, remind yourself for whom you are designing the space, and its purpose.

Trust yourself and your instincts. You know your child better than anyone else.

Chapter 3:

Understanding and Selecting Color

Color is the most important design decision when attempting to elicit an emotional response. It is the primary factor for creating a specific atmosphere. When choosing colors, you must carefully reflect on the result you wish to achieve.

We are all very affected by the colors that surround us. For children, the affects are more palpable. Children, in general, are more sensitive, more observant, and more responsive to sensory information. With special needs and autistic children, the effects can be magnified to the extreme. Children need to be in a surrounding that speaks to their individual needs. Parents and teachers often assume that colorful, playful décor is appropriate for all children. Unfortunately, this is very often not the case.

For centuries, color and its effects on emotion have been recognized and studied. The fact that different colors tend to elicit specific emotional responses has not been overlooked by the government or the medical industry. For example, schools, hospitals, military facilities and prisons have frequently been designed with specific colors in order to influence mood and behavior. Soft, cool blues and greens are extremely common in these environments, because they tend to have a soothing effect. The same principles work just as well in less institutional applications.

As a parent, you may say, *"My child's just an infant or toddler, how can I really know what kind of décor would be best? Could it really have a substantial impact at such a young age?"* Children are like sponges for all types of sensory input. We often don't think much of the things our young children see, are surrounded by, hear, or are exposed to. We make the mistake of assuming that they won't notice or remember, but before we know it, they're mimicking words or behaviors and learning things we didn't anticipate. Babies and toddlers are more in tune with their environments than you might think, and absorb more sensory input than most adults.

Once you have taken into account your child's unique needs, and are aware that color is profoundly important to their environment, you're ready to start the color selection process. Many people become overwhelmed with all the choices available. There are infinite hues and shades, and the differences between many are very subtle. It's difficult enough to evaluate them when they're on a small sample card, but in reality, when they're covering an entire wall, they often look and feel entirely different.

In order to make the "right" selections, start by clarifying your goals. Whom is this room for? How do I want them to feel in the space? How will the room be used? Is it for work or play? Activity, relaxation, or a combination of purposes? Your choices should not only be about what colors go well together, what may be popular or trendy or what sells the best, particularly when there is a special needs child involved. Color selection is intensely subjective and personal. Many of us leave it up to someone else simply because they may have "great taste." Good taste is helpful, but one must really understand the needs of the child and their family. Again these things are entirely individual.

Once you are completely clear on the desired effect of the room based on the child's individual needs, you can begin narrowing down the appropriate colors, or you can convey your goals to a design specialist who can assist you in navigating through the wealth of options on hand. Utilizing a third party can be helpful, but when working with autistic and other special needs children, you need to be the guiding light behind every choice. Nobody will understand your child better than you do.

The following guide provides a general overview of various colors and the emotional responses they typically elicit in neuro-typical individuals. Remember, responses will not be the same for everybody. Many people physically interpret colors differently. For example, there are several different common types of color blindness (more common in men than women). However, these guidelines will be effective more often than not.

Red is the color of blood, heat and fire (an orange based red). It is typically associated with energy, war, danger, strength, power and determination, as well as passion, desire, and love. It tends to stimulate energy and sometimes aggression. Red also tends to evoke feelings of hostility. It should not be used as the main color of a room. It will have a tendency to break down any peace and harmony you are striving to create in your home. Be aware that orange-based reds often correspond to desire, sexual passion, pleasure, domination and thirst for action. Use with care! These are much brighter and visually stimulating, such as a fire engine red. Blue-based reds, like a brick red or burgundy, are warmer and subtle in appearance providing a much cozier feel.

Dark Red is associated with vigor, will-power, rage, anger, leadership, courage, longing, malice, wrath and power. Dark red also energizes and invigorates. It exudes confidence. It can be very helpful in supporting those who are exceedingly withdrawn or exhibit profound lethargy. However, it can also add proverbial fuel to the fire if it surrounds an individual with a hot temper or anger issues. Deep, dark reds that have a blue base rather than an orange base can be great as an accent color to a warm earth tone such as brown.

Light Red represents joy, sensuality, passion, sensitivity, and love. These less intense versions of red can elicit a combination of feelings such as warmth and security, romance, joy, and feelings of sustained energy. Conversely, it can also tend to irritate and agitate as well. So it might be best to confine it to the smaller accessories meant to compliment the space.

Yellow is associated with sunshine, joy, happiness, intellect and energy. Many parents choose yellow for their children's rooms thinking it will be "cheery", but use with caution. It is an uplifting and energizing color, but can sometimes be too much, particularly for a special needs child. People are more likely to lose their tempers, and some parents have observed that their babies tend to cry more, in a yellow room. This color tends to create feelings of frustration and anger in some people, and can be fatiguing on the eyes. It's best to utilize yellow in smaller amounts if you like the brighter more primary tones. If more pastel or subtle shades of yellow are your preference, consider contrasting it with cooler colors for a more tranquil effect. Lighter Yellows are more associated with intellect, freshness, and joy.

Orange combines the energy of red and the happiness of yellow. It is associated with joy, sunshine, and the tropics. Orange represents enthusiasm, fascination, happiness, creativity, determination, attraction, success and encouragement. Remember that it is a stimulating color, and should be used sparingly. Deeper oranges, like rust or cinnamon, which have a browner base, are best when used as a contrasting in a room of neutral warm tones.

Yellow-Green can indicate sickness, cowardice, discord, and jealousy. However, depending on the balance of green to yellow, its effects can vary significantly.

Green is the color of nature. It symbolizes growth, harmony and freshness. Green has a strong emotional correspondence with safety. Many shades of green are cool and soothing and have a calming effect when used as a main color for almost any type of design. It is also believed to relieve stress. Research has found that green can help improve reading ability; by placing a sheet of light green transparency paper over a page in a book, those tested often exhibited increased reading speed and comprehension. Those with varying degrees of dyslexia were also noted as showing major improvement as well. Moss Green is the traditional color of balance and is an example of a "middle of the road" shade of green. It is typically very calming, and emulates the surrounding colors of nature.

Dark Green is traditionally associated with ambition, greed, and jealousy. However, its emotional impact tends to be somewhat different. It tends to have a calming effect and is believed to relieve stress. Darker greens, however, absorb a great deal of light and can inadvertently make a room much darker than intended. It reduces the energy of a space if used on too large a scale.

Blue, the color of the sky and sea is often associated with depth and stability. It symbolizes trust, loyalty, wisdom, confidence, intelligence, faith, truth, and heaven. Like green, it is a cool, soothing color in general. Blue is known to have a calming effect when used as the main color of a room, especially in softer shades.

Light Blue is associated with health, healing, tranquility, understanding, and softness. It's wonderful both as a main color and a contrasting color.

Dark Blue represents knowledge, power, integrity, and seriousness. Dark blue can have the opposite effect of light blue. It often evokes feelings of sadness. One should typically refrain from using darker blues as the dominant color in a space. Stay with the lighter shades of blue to provide a soothing effect. Add darker blues as more of an accent or contrasting color.

Turquoise is associated with emotional healing and protection. However, a very bright shade can be overly stimulating, so once again, use it sparingly unless the purpose of the space it to provide stimulation or a high level of sustained energy. A softer, more muted version can be much less overwhelming to the senses.

Purple combines the stability of blue and the energy of red. Purple is a traditional color of royalty. It symbolizes power, nobility, luxury, and ambition. It conveys wealth and extravagance. Purple is also associated with wisdom, dignity, independence, creativity, mystery, and magic. In terms of design, purple can be used as a "middle of the road" color, but if it's a pure purple, like violet (which is typically on the darker side) it's best to use as a complimentary color or as an accent wall. The other walls should be a cooler, lighter shade, such as a subtle gray or lighter shade of purple. Combining other bright, bold colors with purple, like red, will create an immense amount of stimulation and high energy.

Light Purple evokes romantic and nostalgic feelings. Shades like lilac and lavender can be very soothing especially when paired with similar shades, like other soft blues that combine purples in the base, such as perrywinkle. Light purples are often effective as the overall color of a space that requires tranquility without draining one's energy.

Dark Purple, like eggplant, can often evoke gloom and sad feelings when surrounded by it continually. It can cause frustration if overly used.

White is the presence of all colors. It is associated with light, goodness, innocence and purity. It is considered to be the color of perfection. In a room, white tends to be harsh and stark. It reflects so much light that it can be overwhelming. It is rarely a good choice for children or the elderly as the starkness can create anxiety and aggression, so be forewarned. Breaking it up with another contrasting color will make a huge difference! White can make a room appear spacious but it can also make the room seem unfriendly. When using white as a main color, add color accents in the room to lend a warm and inviting touch. White can also be described as cold and bland. Hospitals often use white to create a sense of sterility, so if you decide on white for a larger area, look for whites that add a touch of cream or neutral to the base – the difference will be visceral to those spending any amount of prolonged time within the room.

While white is often used to create the feeling of a clean, pure, and wholesome space commercially, if the white selected is too bright, it can have a very negative effect. This is why your choice of lighting is also so integral to the feel of a space, as the way if effects the wall color can dramatically change the look of the color and feel of the room.

Black is the absence of all color. It is associated with power, elegance, formality, death, evil, and mystery. It would be extremely unusual for someone to choose black as the primary color for a bedroom. Black, on its own, can exacerbate feelings of negativity and depression. Black in combination with white, stainless steel, pewter, or certain types of wood, can achieve a modern, minimalist look that doesn't necessarily evoke a negative emotional response.

Rather, it's more an expression of personal style. When designing for special needs children, it may not help achieve any particular purpose.

Gray often has negative connotations and is associated with aging or withering. However, gray is also known as a professional color, and though it may seem cold or austere in certain settings, it is often interpreted as classic, denoting wealth and modernism. It also tends to establish a minimalistic sense of personal expression and style, depending on how it's utilized within the design. It's also a wonderful choice when contrasting a bolder color against it as it's not as severe as black and can work with almost any color (note the "*almost*"!)

***

Studies have shown that a person's cultural background and traditions influence their response to color as well. For example some Middle Eastern countries view blue as protective and paint their front doors various shades of blue to ward off evil spirits. Some Asian cultures believe that a red front door draws positive energy into the home and indicates prosperity and purple can eventually draw one to wealth. Be aware that cultural influences can affect how we perceive color, but these are learned over time and should not be allowed to affect decision-making regarding your children's environments.

Another important thing to remember is that while we've addressed some of the basic colors on the color wheel, there are infinite hues that can create completely different emotional responses. The following are some more examples, and the emotions commonly associated with them.

Pink signifies romance, love, and friendship. It often denotes feminine qualities and passiveness. It inspires compassion. It can also help induce a meditative state. Surrounding oneself with pink can encourage feelings of happiness and the sense of being loved, which leads to an improved sense of security.

Brown suggests stability and denotes masculine qualities. Although brown may seem like a depressing color, it's often used as a versatile neutral that works perfectly as a contrast to many different colors. It's also very warm and often provides an intensely "cozy" feeling. Brown is an earth tone, like green, and represents growth and fertility, healing and protection. It is a grounding shade that provides a sense of balance. Consider the look of natural woods; the variations of colors and shades available, whether in paint, stains or natural woods. Brown, and all its variations, offer an authentic "outdoorsy" feel.

Red-Brown is associated with harvest and fall. This particular color combines the energy and warmth of both red and brown, so combining it with darker hues of either color can work well in a room, especially if used with rich dark woods like cherry or walnut. Red-Brown offers a feeling of renewal and plenty. It can spur the desire to begin a new project or job…a change. Subliminally, it's often very motivating due to the bright rich colors produced by nature.

This information can be somewhat overwhelming, and while it can help you make better decisions, it can also be confusing. The purpose of this overview is to illuminate some common assumptions and offer a point of reference from which to begin making your personal selections. Remember, this is a smattering of examples from an infinite array of choices.

Chapter 4:

How to Deal with Multi-Purpose Spaces

Every room in your home has a specific purpose. When we move into a new home, we quickly determine the purpose of each room. In some cases, this decision is made for us by the architectural design. In other cases, it's up to our imagination. Frequently we have very specific ideas about the purpose of each room, how we want it to look, and how we want to feel once we're spending time there. However, there are times that necessity demands we use a room for more than one purpose.

Unexpectedly, our private office doubles as a playroom for the kids, or the master bedroom doubles as a nursery. Before you know it, you're buried in clutter and cannot effectively focus on work, decompress or relax. You fall behind in your work and can't begin to deal with the mere idea of cleaning up the mess even though you know it's essential.

You will need to make compromises. It's important to adapt to the unexpected. Regardless of whether things work out exactly as you planned or not, once the purpose of the room has been determined, it's imperative you acknowledge it and design accordingly.

These questions should act as your guide.

1. How do you create a space that can provide for more than one need?
2. How do you ensure that it will suit both its primary purpose and its secondary needs?

3. Most importantly, regardless of the room's intended use, how do you choose a color and design that won't be distracting or inappropriate for either concern?

Your first thought should be the individual needs of your children. What type of support do they need? Next, determine your needs as parents and caregivers. Finally, think about the overall needs of the family unit. Once these questions have been clearly answered, it will be easier to move forward.

Identifying your space gives you permission to behave a certain way and establishes what you need to accomplish in that space. We unconsciously align ourselves mentally, physically and emotionally even before we take one step into a room, based solely on its designated purpose.

Every design element you choose for a room, from color to furnishings to accents, should align with the purpose of that room. It's very important to maintain the integrity of the space, and to arrange all the visual and sensory stimuli to suit the room's purpose.

Some of the more conventional room combinations tend to be home office/playroom, master bedroom/nursery and family room/playroom. While these combinations are often a necessity to save space, they also create clutter, visual chaos and a huge lack of organization. Subsequently, they can generate anxiety and moodiness within the household. The good news is that there are several simple ways to minimize and in some cases eliminate these somewhat minor issues. Don't procrastinate; if you ignore the problem, it will more than likely grow worse.

Begin by looking at subtle or neutral paint colors so that energy can be maintained rather than increased or drained when spending a prolonged amount of time in the space.

Some examples include Café Au Lait, Mocha, Almond, Lavender, Sea-Foam Green or Glacier Blue. These shades are less intrusive and promote more focused attention over a longer period of time. In general, the deeper and earthier the tone, the warmer and "cozier" it becomes. The cooler the color, the more pacifying it tends to be.

The most effective way to provide structure and avoid conflict is to create a schedule for the use of the room. As an example, kids have playtime from 10am until noon. Then it becomes a home office from noon until 3pm. Of course, not everything works out that smoothly. It takes patience and effort to stick to a schedule.

To keep the purposes of the space from encroaching upon one another, utilize storage units, such as drawers or cabinets, that are opaque (in other words, *not* transparent). This is extremely helpful in reducing temptation for children as well as avoiding visual overload for everyone sharing the space. Belongings can be kept in their proper place until it's appropriate to use them.

Mobile wall divisions, such as Chinese screens, are wonderfully decorative and often inexpensive ways to create separation and privacy within the space. It is often possible to organize the room in such a way that different parts of the space are designated for specific purposes. If you can do this whenever possible, it will help minimize intrusions and distractions.

Remember, autistic children usually depend on regimented and consistent schedules. Routine is very important to their sense of well-being and security. Setting a schedule and dividing the space effectively can be the ideal way to support their needs as well as your own.

Chapter 5:

Avoiding Common Mistakes

There are several potential pitfalls one can encounter when determining the décor for children's rooms. The most common is probably the traditional tendency to be attached to color based on gender:

Pink for girls, Blue for boys.

While many parents have begun to break that tendency, it still seems to be the common basis for design in children's rooms. There is nothing inherently wrong with selecting colors based on gender; the problem is related more to the shades so often selected and the assumption that gender is the *only* consideration necessary when determining your child's color scheme. Remember, the way a neuro-typical child responds to primary and/or bright colors may be vastly different than the way a special needs child might respond. Using softer versions of these colors may be fine, but again, it's important to bear in mind how they're used.

Just remember that gender is generally not one of the more important considerations when selecting colors. Understand your child's individual needs and select colors accordingly. For instance, an "upbeat" bright pink may seem like the perfect idea for your sweet five year-old little girl. She may like the color, but she doesn't recognize that it can be the cause of a great deal of agitation, and an inability to relax or focus; an overall feeling of chaos she's unable to convey. This reaction could manifest in the form of prolonged negative behavior. She may be consistently upset or frustrated, unable to sleep in her room and could even act out physically. The neuro-typical child might have a similar reaction, though it's rare that the response would be this extreme.

Another consideration is the ceiling. Should you leave it as is? Give it color? Do you paint a sky line with clouds or an outer space motif with planets and stars? Or do you paint it a solid color? If so, should it be darker or lighter than the wall colors? Should you hang educational mobiles depending on your child's age or cognitive needs? Just like the aforementioned examples, you must take into account all the specific challenges your child presently encounters and what your goals are for them. Then it will be much easier to arrive at a conclusion. The common mistake is to choose what you think will be "cool" or "fun" without first taking time to consider the greater impact it may have on your child.

The challenge here is that results tend to vary quite a bit from child to child. It's helpful to learn about other parents' experiences, but not count on their experiences or results to be the same for your child no matter what the children's similarities might be. A general rule with any design on a ceiling is to focus on the size of the room. Darker colors tend to make the room feel smaller and lighter colors open it up and allow for a more spacious feel. This is the best guideline to use when deliberating over your design. Think about the goals you have for your child's environment and choose accordingly. Remember, you can always change it later. All you need is a paint brush.

You may have noticed that clutter can exacerbate your child's sense of turmoil and chaos. After all, it tends to affect all of us the same way. However, as already explained, its effects are much more visceral for the special needs/autistic child. When deciding how to store your child's books, toys and games, one common mistake is to use open shelves or large, clear plastic bins. It might seem like the perfect solution due to the fact that you can see where everything is, and find particular items quickly. However, exposing all these objects, all the various colors and shapes, tends to create an overload of visual stimulation which can once again, increase anxiety and create distractions.

Instead of open or clear storage units, look for options that utilize closed cabinets or opaque drawers. That way everything can be put away and remain out of sight. The visual overload is averted. You can select what you want to remain in sight and what should be stored away until the appropriate time for it to be used. There are some things you may want to put on shelves, but these should be selected carefully based on importance and frequency of use. Try to keep them to a minimum.

One final inclination to avoid is over-filling the room. People have a tendency to occupy every inch of available space. Smaller rooms are typically easy to arrange, because often there's only so much you can do. Larger rooms, however, offer more choices. You should resist the temptation to utilize every conceivable piece of furniture in hopes of making the room seem less empty. Space can be a good thing; less really *is* more.

In short, take some time to alter the way you think about décor. Focus on the goals you have for your child within their personal space. Utilizing these principles and guidelines should make creating the perfect environment for *your* child a much easier more enjoyable endeavor.

***

The following is a real-life example of the pitfalls parents fall into that can often create an immediate negative reaction in their child, yet can still easily go unnoticed.

My friend Cheryl was sharing the excitement she felt for her nephew Henry, as he had just turned three years old. Her sister and brother-in-law had just re-decorated his room. They sent her pictures and told her how impressed the neighbors were with their "cool" new design.

All the walls were white with bright primary colors splashed all around the room. Two big red bean bag chairs, shelves filled with toys and books, a small television for movies, white shades with colored polka-dots, and a brightly colored throw rug adorned the space. It sounded tremendously fun and kid friendly. What Cheryl's sister didn't know was that her young son Henry was getting out of his bed every night and walking down the hall to sleep in Daddy's office.

It took her three days to realize that Henry wasn't sleeping through the night in his own bed. Henry was an early riser, so the problem went unnoticed at first. Apparently, the lack of sleep was catching up with him. She went to his room to check on him one morning, but instead, found him fast asleep on Dad's office floor. Apparently little Henry was so anxiety ridden by the colors and design of his room that he decided to go elsewhere. His father's office was a neutral light brown, and a light, fresh blue with darker brown wood. It had soft white natural light and two large floor plants.

The remarkable thing is that instead of crying, acting out, or simply going to his parents' room as most children would, Henry instinctively knew where to go in his home to find peace and comfort. Autistic children often respond to situations like this in surprising ways.

It doesn't take much to see the obvious differences when compared side by side, yet while Henry's room was clearly aesthetically "fun" and age appropriate, it was completely *inappropriate* for Henry. There are ways to accomplish both a feeling of fun and supportive tranquility. That's our goal.

Children can't always describe what they're feeling or experiencing, but they react to their needs in the only way they are able. In this case, Henry needed more tranquil surroundings in order to rest. It's important to know what to look for and to pay close attention.

Chapter 6:

It's Easy Being "Green"

Before you do anything, consider the materials you choose. Paint is the first concern. Many of the most popular brands have good coverage, a wide range of colors and great longevity. However, many paints are somewhat toxic. The unpleasant smell of fresh paint is a warning sign. The fumes they emit are unhealthy. Have you ever planned for open windows or overnights at friends' homes hoping to "air out" the room, or your whole house? You may think that when the odor fades, everything is OK. However, while the scent may dissipate, the chemicals that are released into the air can continue to affect you for years.

Some of the most dangerous culprits are VOC's (volatile organic compounds). There are numerous types of VOC's and they can cause a variety of different health issues depending on the amount of the exposure and the length of exposure. Awareness of the problem has grown to the point that the paint industry has finally begun to react and take positive action.

Now that going "green" has become both a necessity and a trend, many household companies have given in and become part of the wave of environmental consciousness. As consumers, we can now take full advantage of the "green" trend and acquire healthier paints for our homes. There are many companies that have removed or are in process of removing VOC's from their paint, and these paints are not hard to find. They do cost more, but isn't the health of your family worth it?

With a Brush of Love doesn't officially endorse any particular manufacturer, but we have several recommendations based on our experience.

Benjamin Moore has two brands of low or zero VOC paint: *Natura* and *Aura Guard*. *Natura* was scheduled to be available nation-wide in the Spring of 2009, and may already be available in your area. It exceeds the criteria for environmental safety set forth by *LEED* (Leadership in Energy and Environmental Design) & Green Seal GS-11 standards. It is very smooth and easy to apply, has great coverage, color selection and is fairly cost effective. It adheres very well and has excellent longevity.

FreshAire Choice is another quality brand to consider. At this time, both *Aura Guard* and *FreshAire Choice* can be found at Home Depot. *Natura* is still only available at Benjamin Moore dealers or online. While *Natura* is a VOC free paint, both *FreshAire Choice* and *Aura Guard* are very low in VOC's and are viable alternatives. While VOC's are bad for all of us, they can be especially harmful to special needs children and those with autism. Much in the same way they are more sensitive to foods, special needs children tend to react more intensely to chemical exposure. Your paint choice is much more than simply picking your children's favorite colors.

Another way to "go green" is to take the expression literally. Plants are a great addition to almost any room, and they have several significant benefits, both physically and psychologically. Try to consciously perceive your reaction when you enter a new space that has plants, as opposed to one that does not. The difference can be quite extreme. Under normal circumstances you may not notice why you may feel differently, but the impact is tangible.

There are several different types of plants that are easy to care for and preferable for those children with sensory issues.

One of the things that make them so beneficial is that they filter the air naturally.

Several plants, some of which are shown below, were included by NASA in their Clean Air Study, which researched various ways to clean air in space stations. In addition to absorbing carbon dioxide and releasing oxygen, as all plants do, these plants also eliminate significant amounts of benzene, formaldehyde and/or trichloroethylene, a natural filtering process of the plant and an important plus for all sensitive individuals, especially children with sensitive health and overall respiratory issues.

Some of these plants include:

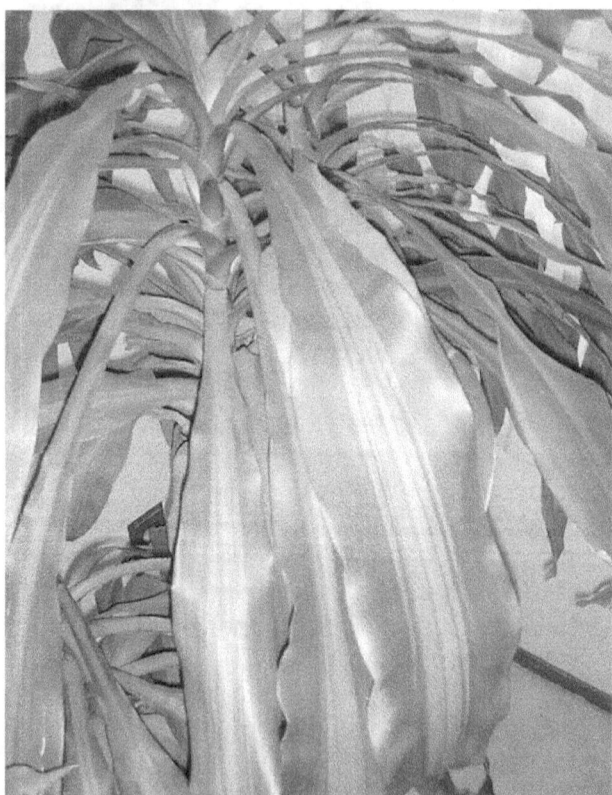

Cornstalk Dracaena

Peace Lily (Spathiphyllum)

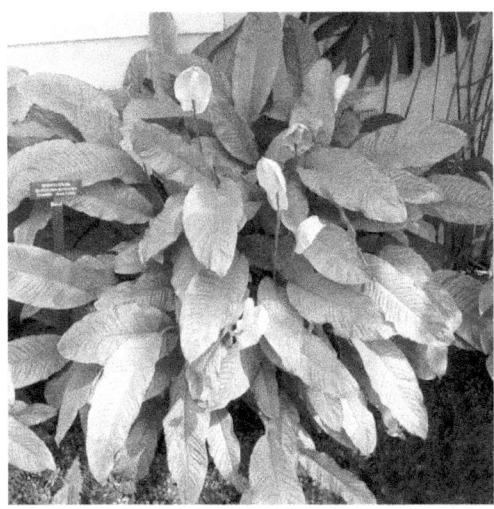 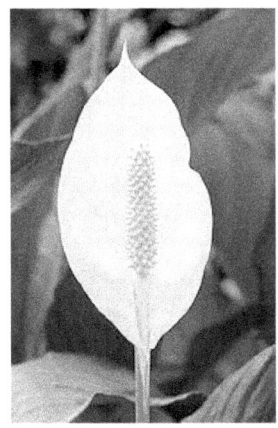

Chrysanthemum

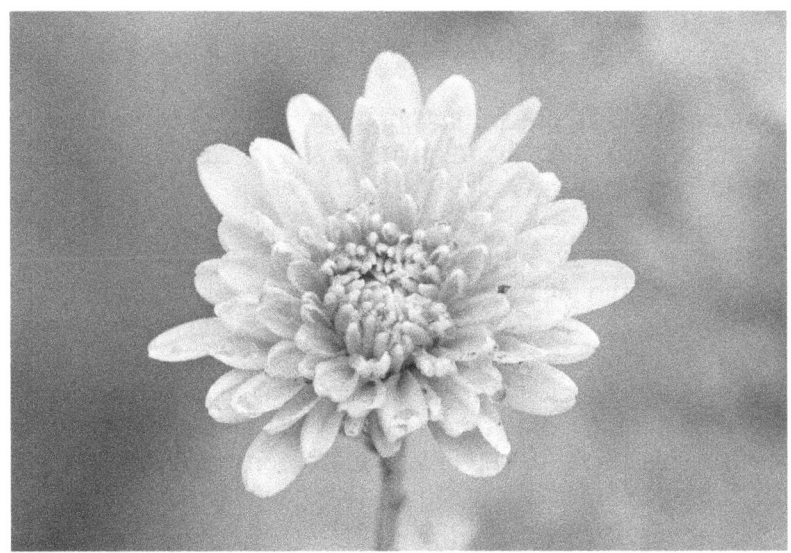

Gerbera

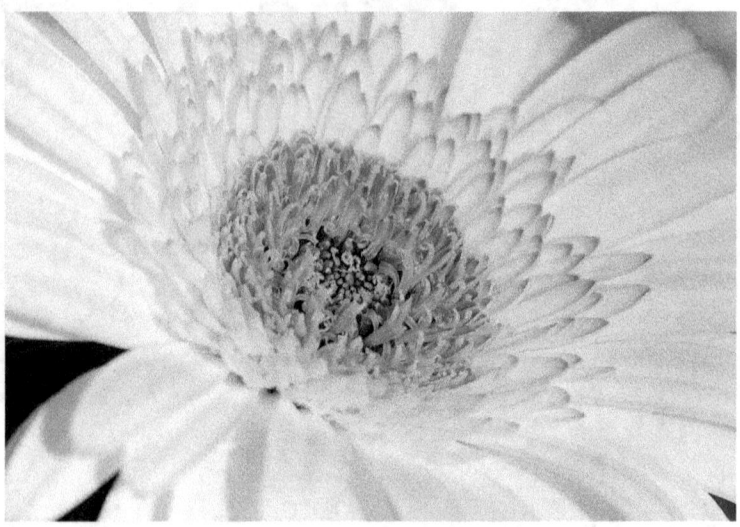

For a full list of these plants, check out:
http://en.wikipedia.org/wiki/List_of_air-filtering_plants

Another trend in "green" design is lighting. This applies not just to energy savings and environmental protection, but to health and safety as well.

Mercury is a heavy metal associated with contamination of water, fish, and food supplies. There are many dangers of mercury poisoning. A CFL bulb generally contains an average of 5 mg of mercury (about one-fifth of that found in the average watch battery, and less than 1/100th of the mercury found in an amalgam dental filling). In order to generate the amount of power needed to light a standard incandescent bulb, a power plant will emit approximately 10 mg of mercury. This compares to only 2.4mg of mercury to run a CFL bulb for the same amount of time. The net benefit of using the more energy efficient lamp is positive, and this is especially true if the mercury in the fluorescent lamp is kept out of the waste stream when the lamp expires.

All fluorescent lamps do not contain the same amount of mercury. Philips lamps with Alto Lamp Technology, for instance, contain less mercury than conventional fluorescent lamps. Philips claims the bulbs have the lowest amount of mercury of any bulb on the market at less than 3.8 mg per bulb. While having mercury in the light bulbs in your child's room isn't immediately hazardous, it could become so if that bulb breaks.

If you break one:

- open a window and leave the room for 15 minutes or more
- use a wet rag to clean it up and put all of the pieces, and the rag, into a plastic bag
- place all materials in a second sealed plastic bag
- call your local recycling center to see if they accept this material, otherwise put it in your local trash. Wash your hands afterward.

Burned out CFLs can be dropped off at Home Depot and Ikea stores for disposal. Another solution is to save spent CFLs for a community household hazardous waste collection, which would then send the bulbs to facilities capable of treating, recovering or recycling them. For more information on CFL disposal or recycling, you can contact your local municipality.

An alternative to CFL's is LED (Light Emitting Diode) bulbs. These are small, solid light bulbs that are extremely energy-efficient. Until recently, LEDs were relegated primarily to industrial uses. They can be seen in instrument panels, electronics, pen lights and, more recently, strings of indoor and outdoor Christmas lights. On a grander scale, however, they are used to create enormous video displays, bright enough to be seen in full daylight (stadium video scoreboards, for example). These are made of thousands of colored LEDs that, in combination, create one large video image. The vast improvement in the brightness and efficiency of LEDs has resulted in their use in flashlights and light bulbs.

Many different models and styles of LED bulbs are becoming available as safe, energy efficient alternatives to incandescent bulbs and CFL's. In order to select the right one, use the same considerations as with any bulbs:

- Desired wattage - a 3W LED is equivalent in output to a 45 W incandescent.
- Warm vs. cool light - new LED bulbs are available in 'cool' white light, which is ideal for task lighting, and 'warm' light commonly used for accent or small area lighting.
- Standard base or pin base - LEDs are available in several types of pin sockets or the standard screw (Edison) bases for recessed or track lighting.

The common styles of LED bulbs are:

Recessed/Track bulbs - Available in pin base or standard (Edison) base, LEDs are ideal for track or recessed lighting. LEDs do not contribute to heat buildup in a room because no matter how long they remain on, they do not get hot to the touch. Also, because they are 90% more efficient than incandescent, the frequency of changing bulbs is greatly reduced.

Diffused bulbs

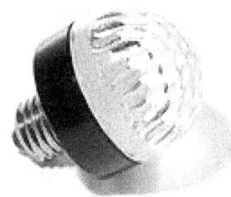

In this style LED bulb, clusters of LEDs are covered by a dimpled lens which spreads the light out over a wider area. Available in a range of wattage and sizes, these bulbs have many uses, such as area lighting for small rooms, porches, reading lamps, accent lamps, hallways and low-light applications where lights remain on for extended periods.

Spotlight and Floodlight LEDs

The spotlight LED lacks a dispersing lens, so it appears brighter as its light is directed forward. The floodlight model gives a spread-out dispersed light. Well suited for ceiling lights, outdoor floodlights, retail display lighting, landscape lighting and motion sensors.

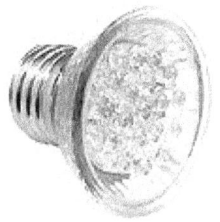

Chapter 7:

Spatial Organization

Once you've selected your color palette and have begun to understand the needs of your child, it will be easier to translate what furniture/storage items are necessary to organize your child's environment.

First and foremost, determine what is actually necessary within the space. Do not simply choose furniture in order to keep the room from feeling empty. The size of the room is obviously of prime consideration. However, just because it may be larger, it doesn't mean you need to fill the open space with unnecessary furniture.

Here are some questions to consider before you purchase any new items or make any significant changes:

1. How much furniture will the room realistically accommodate?
2. What types of specific concerns need to be met? (i.e. home therapy sessions, playtime, sharing with siblings)
3. Are the furniture items you're considering functional or are they more design oriented?
4. Are the storage components compatible with your needs or do they take up space while leaving you with organizational and/or clutter concerns?

Answering these questions honestly will help make your decisions much more obvious. However, once you've narrowed down which pieces of furniture you want, there's the issue of how they should be placed within the room. Some rooms don't allow for many options due to the placement of doors, closets and windows, but there are usually more options than you might think. It just takes some creative planning and a bit of patience.

Most of us make visual assumptions about where certain types of furniture should be placed. However, there really aren't any rules. For example, many people tend to place sofas, chairs and ottomans (any variation of seating) in the center of a room facing one another thinking it will create cozy intimacy for guests. If this same tendency is applied to a bedroom, the room may feel closed-off or cluttered. This is particularly true of smaller rooms, which can easily start to feel claustrophobic. Most people don't realize that the placement of furniture is often the primary cause of the frustration they feel in a particular space.

A small room doesn't necessarily need to *feel* small or even look small. There are many ways to place furniture. For example, don't assume you should place the bed with the head against the wall forcing it into the heart of the room. Rather, consider turning it sideways placing it somewhat "flush" against the wall, taking advantage of the wall space. It is not always the best solution, or even the preferred choice of placement; it's ultimately dependent upon the size of the selected items and the layout of the room. The point is, consider various possibilities before making a decision. There are often more options for placement and organization than you might realize if you think outside that well known "box."

If you're going to put a piece of furniture in a corner, try to place it as close to the corner as possible. Perhaps try a "caddy corner" position, diagonal toward the center of the room. The size of the piece will determine how well this will work.

The open space should ideally "flow", not just in a "feng shui" way, but rather like a clear pathway allowing for easy access to all areas. Nothing should feel closed off simply due to the location of a dresser or a desk.

Again, there are no hard and fast rules about how to place furniture. In some cases you may want to turn a bed with its head against the wall, or place a chair away from a corner leaving a path around the perimeter of the room. The key is to make sure there is a "flow", and to not close off areas in such a way that you have to walk around things to get to them.

As previously mentioned, avoid utilizing clear plastic tubs and containers for storing children's items. Again, while they may make it easier to find things or quickly determine where they belong, they do nothing to hide the myriad of colors and shapes of the objects they contain. They visual chaos and complexity can over-stimulate special needs children. This can cause agitation, hinder their ability to focus, and in general, undermine your effort to create a tranquil, supportive environment for everyone.

Closed storage units, such as drawers, cabinets with opaque doors, or solid colored containers, tend to work much better. Your children only see the items when it's time to use them, avoiding temptation and distraction. Each storage area is like a "station", to be utilized as needed. Otherwise, it remains closed and the visual stimulation is avoided. Autistic children rely heavily on consistency, stability and a sense of order. These guidelines can actually assist in addressing all these concerns as well as assisting the children to follow the guidelines and rules you wish to establish.

Chapter 8:

Images, Patterns and Designs

People tend to operate under the misconception that other people have the same tastes and preferences they do. When you go shopping for a gift, how often do you pick something because it appeals to *you*, without having a full understanding of the person for whom you're buying it? Have you ever found out, after the fact, that your selection was completely wrong? This works both ways, of course. Perhaps someone whom you believe knows you very well gave you a gift that didn't suit you at all. Perhaps it was the pattern, design, or overall style that didn't appeal to you.

Patterns and designs are just as subjective as colors. The reasons we tend to favor specific lines, colors, styles and patterns are very personal, and are typically related to our individual experiences and our personalities.

Patterns can be tiny, providing a "textured" look, particularly when viewed at a distance (like a hounds-tooth). They can also be large and clearly defined. Patterns, like art, are also very subjective, and people respond in different ways. It is also important to remember that if your child says he or she "loves" a pattern, it does not mean that using it in his/her room is a good idea. Attraction to a pattern does *not* automatically translate on a grand scale. It's the emotional and psychological reaction over a long period of exposure that matters.

Semantics can be challenging when discussing this concept, so let's take a moment to clarify the distinction between a "design" and a "pattern." A design is contained, or finite. It occupies a confined space. A pattern is continuous. The designer, in this case, you, should distinguish the difference and consider the intricacies (or lack thereof) in either a pattern or design to which your child may gravitate.

The use and selection of images are very important as they can make a substantial impression on a child, both consciously and subliminally. Consider the image of a clown. In the context of a circus, clowns are playful and fun. The imagery of a circus is very specific: animals, a ringmaster, balloons, trapeze artists, etc. Out of this context, the image of a clown may have a completely different impact. Clown figurines displayed on a shelf at night can be creepy or haunting. How many children are terrified of clowns at birthday parties? There are even adults who are uncomfortable with, or afraid of clowns. Be very careful of the images you choose. Consider how your child may react under various circumstances. Not every child-like image, regardless of how benign it may seem, is appropriate to use in your child's surroundings.

While the idea of brightly colored rockets, large zoo animals, or "fun" primary colors may seem to be perfect for your child's décor, they may ultimately do more harm than good. What your child sees can be wildly different from what you anticipate. Bright, bold images can become very ominous and overwhelming to some children, leading to unnecessary anxiety, insecurity, trepidation or even fear. There is no absolute rule for every autistic child, but you must get to know your child in ways he or she may not communicate to you verbally or directly. If you even suspect they may react negatively, avoid those images, at least at first. Test the waters, and don't integrate these images into your design until you are certain of how your child will respond.

These guidelines don't come without options. There is no need to completely disappoint a child by saying "no" to including a design, pattern or image they're drawn to. Here is a compromise you can offer:

1. Cut out a small sample of the desired pattern, design or image. Measure it, matte and frame it as you would a photo. Keep it small enough to place on a bedside table or nearby dresser at eye level. This way your child is satisfied and sees that their request has been acknowledged. It's important that they know you're listening.

2. Keep the frame a solid color: wood, silver, pewter, aluminum or plastic. As a general rule, avoid bright colors and patterns. Frames should also remain somewhat small. This way the image requested remains contained. If, however, your child loves a particularly bright color, you can utilize it as the solid color of a standing frame or lamp shade, but keep it small.

3. Minimize the number of frames in order to avoid visual clutter. Try to use no more than three frames at eye level and two to three on the walls. Keep in mind the size of the space when determining the appropriate amount.

Photos of family members, particularly parents, should be used in at least two to three of the total framed items, as it provides a sense of security for the child. One of the most common challenges parents face with special needs children is getting them to become comfortable sleeping in their own room. Photos of family members (including themselves) help to ease separation anxiety. They help children remain in their own space without feeling completely alone or isolated from Mom and Dad.

With these helpful hints, you should now feel free to begin personalizing your design. Just don't forget to have FUN!

Chapter 9:

Shared Bedrooms

If you grew up with a sibling, you may be one of the many who shared a bedroom. There are several compromises children must make in this situation. They must learn to cooperate, share and adapt in one space together. This is not an easy task regardless of how well siblings may get along.

Figuring out how to combine the likes and dislikes of two completely individual personalities is never easy. When one or both of them have a special need, such as autism, it presents even larger challenges. There is no easy way to answer the question of how to design for this type of scenario, but it always helps to learn from experience. Here's an example of two brothers with different needs in one bedroom.

Envision two brothers around the ages 4 and 7. We'll call them *Robert and Kevin*. Kevin, the younger brother, has Aspergers Syndrome (a high functioning form of autism). Robert is neuro-typical with an abundance of energy. Each has completely opposite interests and tastes. While the brothers seem to get along fairly well, they still experience the normal sibling rivalry. Robert still isn't old enough to understand the unique differences he notices in his little brother and doesn't maintain much tolerance when continually exposed to them.

Robert tends to love lots of bright colors and patterns and an abundance of physical activity. All types of extreme sports, race cars, motorcycles and rockets adorned the walls above Robert's bed. Kevin, on the other hand, likes games and watching videos. He doesn't have much interest in almost any of the things his brother likes. The only thing they really have in common is a talent for mischief!

Kevin tends to fixate on lasers and light sabers from "Star Wars". He gravitates toward softer shades of blue and green whenever given the choice, even when it comes to picking out his school clothes. And of course, they both like watching television. Kevin is much more sensitive than Robert, and becomes agitated very easily. He rarely connects socially with others, and has a tendency to act out physically when he is upset, banging his head against walls or other objects. He needs an environment that is soothing, one that helps him to focus and stay centered.

How did we bring these two brothers together in one room that suited them both? The "how" is always the challenge, but it's also part of the fun!

First and foremost, we selected colors that are calming in nature. When we met Robert and Kevin, their room was painted a vibrant mango-yellow color. Their parents thought it would be cheerful. It was, but it was also entirely over-stimulating. The boys literally bounced off the walls. Kevin had a lot of trouble sleeping, and would regularly make his way to his parents' room at night. That was the first matter that needed to be addressed.

A soothing color would help quell Kevin's tendency toward agitation and mellow Robert as well, making it easier for Kevin to be relaxed around his brother. In this case, the most unobtrusive color that still maintained some energy but didn't overly stimulate was a custom blue that resembles cornflower blue. We cleared out their room, put up a coat of primer, and applied the new color.

The next step was to evaluate their existing furniture. Was it functional? If so, could it be re-finished with stain or paint rather than replaced? In this case, we determined that the best design for them was to replace the furniture, but keep it in a low price range. Furniture selections should be multi-functional, not just aesthetically appealing. Nowadays, it's not hard to find items that accomplish both with all the price points and options available both in stores and on line.

Their original bedroom was over stuffed with furniture that wasn't as functional as it needed to be and cut off the space. There was also clutter and visual chaos everywhere. It was obvious we needed to find furniture that would occupy less space but provide more function by handling the storage needs of both boys. As a result, we would be able to create a more spacious feel.

We found an aluminum bunk bed and two storage units that incorporated adjustable shelving with solid opaque doors. This created both visual and non-visual storage areas so excessive visual stimulation was kept to an absolute minimum. We also found trundle drawers that fit perfectly beneath the bottom bunk, offering two large out of sight areas for storage.

We provided each of the boys with small, personal items that featured their individual interests and requests without encroaching on one another's space. In this case, small pictures and designs on the walls next to their respective bunks or on a small night stand. By keeping certain images contained, we maintained aesthetic control, which was particularly important for Kevin.

We replaced large bulky furniture with light, airy pieces that had twice the functionality and storage capacity. We also re-organized the room by leaving the center clear allowing for an open pathway from one end to the other. Within weeks, the boys' general demeanor changed dramatically. Kevin began sleeping in his room without complaint, and his aggressive tendencies diminished.

This is just one example, but it illustrates how to combine the needs of completely different children without much difficulty. One of the main lessons to be learned is that these design principles are effective for *all* children, not just those with special needs. It's essential to understand the importance of all design elements working together. All the components of a design should fit together like a puzzle in order for the whole room to optimally support and positively affect a child's behaviors and reactions on a daily basis.

Chapter 10:

Use of Other Sensory Elements

The Five Senses: Taste, Touch, Sound, Sight & Smell. These five simple things are what guide us through each day. They act as our personal navigation system. We count on our senses to warn us when something is wrong. They trigger emotions and memories. They determine the foods we like and dislike and what textures we favor. For neuro-typical individuals, senses are a source of information and support in our daily lives. For some however, such as those with autism, the sensory integration doesn't work the same way. The term "sensory overload" is applicable to them on a regular basis. A neuro-typical child generally acclimates to sounds, smells and sights over a period of time. They simply adapt. Those individuals with autism and various other special needs tend to be much more sensitive. The things most of us may simply adapt to can overwhelm them. The effect may apply to all their senses, or it may just be particular ones.

Parents should observe and try to become more keenly aware of which senses affect their children most intensely. It's important to observe both the positives and the negatives. The impacts of various sights, sounds, smells, tastes and textures are critical components of a child's emotional state, especially when trying to decipher what "makes them tick." Depending on the child's age and level of verbal communication, it may not be easy. It takes patient observation as well as basic trial and error to truly familiarize yourself with your child's habits and tendencies.

As you're discovering your child's likes and dislikes, you will probably notice similarities that will help to predict their responses. You may find, for example, that your child likes marbles. What is it about marbles he or she likes? The shape? The texture? The sound they make? The colors? By observing your child's reactions to various objects, you may be able to determine the specific characteristics that they're responding to. Eventually you will be able to use this knowledge as a template and apply it directly.

There are various types of sensory support available: colored fiber optics, bubble makers, aromatherapy, light dimmers and colored gels just to name a few. There's no "right" or "wrong" in terms of how to use them. Nature CD's or sound-scapes like rain, ocean waves (my personal favorite), or birds chirping in the morning can all be ways to help a child or anyone for that matter, relax more fully and assist in replacing internal feelings of anxiety and upset with a sense of inner calm and peacefulness. Even babies are soothed by the simulated sounds of their mother's womb and are easily lulled to sleep when nothing else seems to work. Simplicity is often overlooked and is frequently the ideal solution.

Lighting is a major component of one's atmosphere. Using soft and/or natural light bulbs is very important. Select your lighting carefully. Try to utilize lights with dimmers, or at least multiple brightness settings. Control of both the amount and color of light are important.

Stay away from fluorescent bulbs whenever possible as the color of fluorescent light is simply too harsh for a space that is meant to provide a tranquil atmosphere. If you're looking for an energy saving bulb, do your research, as there are several options on the market to choose from. Refer to Chapter 6 for some suggestions.

None of these are guaranteed solutions. They're simply creative techniques to produce atmospheres that will enhance your child's overall growth and progress.

Chapter 11:

Budget Saving Tips

How do you accomplish everything we've shared on a limited budget? It's not as hard as you might think. Here are some very basic tips:

1. Decide what the most important change should be (paint color, replacing furniture, buying a new bed). Make changes in order of priority. It's not always necessary to do everything at once.
2. Take full advantage of the internet and be "surf savvy," there are loads of search engines that will assist you in finding the information you're looking for. Look for discount stores, estate sales, flea markets and all types of swap meets. Don't ignore second hand stores (thrift shops) as they often have some remarkable finds!
3. Research major shopping websites for simple pieces of furniture. Call them (some even have well-informed salespeople or managers!) Inquire as to when seasonal "floor display" furniture items go on sale. In most home furnishing stores, you can often find discontinued floor items at heavily discounted prices.
4. If you want a new throw rug for your wood or cement floor, but don't want to spend the money, believe it or not, you can create a chic, expensive looking design with paper, pencil, scissors and some paint! Simply enlarge the pattern to the size you desire on a photocopier (just use a sturdy paper) cut out the pattern and viola', instant stencil! Tape it on the area of the floor you want for your design. Get a paintbrush the proper size to fit over the stencil; small enough to work neatly, but no smaller than necessary. Wait a couple of hours and then remove the stencil. It really

does work! Just make sure that the floor material won't repel your paint /stain selection; this process tends to work best on wood and cement.

5. If you want new curtains or window treatments but want to avoid the extra cost, try the do-it-yourself method. Shop at fabric stores for bolts of material or purchase some nice flat bedding sheets. Get an inexpensive curtain rod from a home improvement store and you're on your way. Cut the material to size, wrap it around the curtain rod in any way you want allowing it to hang straight down or use thin strips of any of your favorite material as sashes to tie or knot your curtains to the side. If you're handy with a needle and thread, sewing machine or glue gun, you can add any ornamentation you like for a more personal touch.

6. If you want something resembling a decorative valance, use the aforementioned stenciling process again. It works on walls and moldings too! Just remember to focus on what your child's needs are. It's easy to get caught up trying to be creative and elaborate. The phrase "less is more" couldn't be more appropriate than when designing your child's personal atmosphere.

7. Try taking a swatch of patterned fabric or even gift wrap (yes, attractive wrapping paper) and cut it into a stylized shape. For extra flair, use a patterned scissor. The blades are cut with a unique shape which will create a design in the paper. Then, simply matte and frame as you would any picture or special document. You now have an interesting designer accent for any room. This is particularly useful for providing imagery your child would favor, but would be inappropriate to incorporate on a large scale. Don't underestimate the expensive and original look of such simple design accents, they often become an interesting point of discussion among your many impressed house guests!

These may seem like very simplistic suggestions, however, they are all low cost, artistic, one-of-a-kind, "green" ideas you can use within the design of your child's room as well as your home. Hopefully, you've now begun to understand how to address many of your concerns without feeling overwhelmed or intimidated.

Conclusions

Now that we've discussed how to evaluate your child's needs, understand the purpose of the room you want to re-design, anticipate the effects of various colors, and how to consider spatial organization, my hope is that you feel you have been armed with some fundamental tools that will motivate you to jump on the "do-it-yourself" bandwagon with excitement, and a renewed sense of confidence and control!

These guidelines should help inspire you to be more creative and trust in your own ideas. Employ your imagination and newly acquired knowledge to make a positive change to your child's environment, and subsequently make a significant impact on the quality of their life. When these methods are used to their greatest effect, you may observe a noticeable improvement in the way your child behaves and interacts with you, the rest of your family, and the world around them.

Experiment, observe, learn, and enjoy the process of re-designing your children's space and any other part of your home.

Just remember, no matter what you choose to do, always begin **With a Brush of Love**!

References

Magazine Articles –

- *Life Script: Your Health, Your Life, Your Way*
- *"Tips for Choosing a Room Color Scheme" June 18, 2008*
- *Wikipedia: "Air Filtering Soil & Plants"*
- *Google Search Engine*
- *Earth Easy: "Energy Efficient Lighting"*
- *The New York Times "A Room Comes Alive with Color and Sounds" Dec 23, 2003*
- *Snoezelen : Multi-Sensory Environments*
- *National Review of Medicine : "Have you ever Snoezelened?" January 30,2004*

The photos in this work are published under the following license.

__I, the copyright holder of this work,__ hereby publish it under the following license:

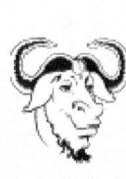

About the Author

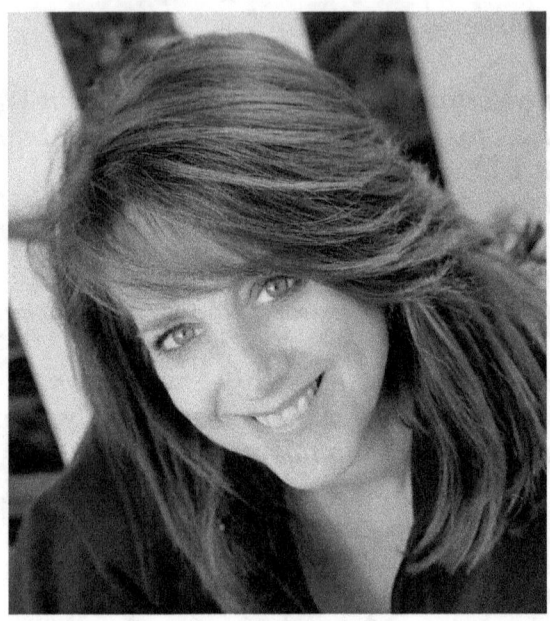

Lauren S. Henry is an experienced children's educator and a veteran of the Montgomery County, MD and Fairfax County, VA school systems. She specializes in the educational and emotional needs of children from pre-kindergarten through sixth grade, as well as those with special needs.

Lauren graduated from Syracuse University's S.I. Newhouse School of Communications and the School of Visual and Performing Arts. In addition, she has, throughout her career, studied child psychology and design. This unique background inspired her to create **With a Brush of Love.**

Lauren thoroughly researched the effects of color on emotion and consulted with psychologists who specialize in this field of study. She has combined this knowledge and her own experience to develop techniques for optimizing the environments of special needs children to provide them the ideal emotional and intellectual support.

As a result of Lauren's work, she has been asked to be a guest designer on HGTV's **kidspace** and ABC television's **Extreme Makeover: Home Edition.** She has also been invited to present to families on the **MCCS Military** base, **Camp Foster** in Okinawa, Japan and the **Exceptional Family Member Program** (designed to assist those military families with special needs children.) She contributes monthly as a columnist for the *Autism at Home Series*.

Lauren currently resides in Los Angeles, California.

For additional information or public relations inquiries, or to arrange guest appearances, speaking engagements or private consultation, visit:

www.brushoflove.com

or email:

lauren@brushoflove.com